Magnesium

The Miracle of Making up Magnesium Deficiency for Women's Health, Relief and Longevity

KARA AIMER

CONTENTS

INTRODUCTION

Magnesium! Many of us have heard about this mineral but do you know how important it is to the body? Are you aware that a deficiency of this essential nutrient can lead to cardiovascular diseases, strokes, and even death in some cases? Magnesium deficiency has even worse consequences in women especially when pregnant.

Do you want to learn more about magnesium and the role this mineral plays in the body? Do you want to know foods that you can eat in order to deal with magnesium deficiency? Are you looking to learn more about the different forms of magnesium available in the market and the best for supplementation? If you are, then this book will give you all the information you need to know about magnesium from the conditions related with magnesium deficiency to ways of addressing it for good.

Magnesium is one of the essential minerals found in the body with half of the mineral being located in the bones. The human body consists of around 25 grams of magnesium, with about 1 percent being found in the blood serum. Magnesium is an important co-factor in at least 300 biochemical reactions in the body. Some of the important functions of magnesium include maintaining optimal functioning of your immune system, regulating the heartbeat, monitoring the nerve function, and building of muscles.

A healthy person should have about 0.75-0.95 mill-moles of magnesium per liter of blood, with the body keeping magnesium levels under tight monitoring. However, serum magnesium levels can drop to less than 0.75 mill-moles per liter, leading to the development of Hypomagnesemia. The kidney controls the level of serum magnesium, by excreting 120 grams of excess magnesium daily through urine. When magnesium level reduces, the excretion is also regulated to ensure the optimum levels are maintained.

FORMS OF MAGNESIUM

Magnesium isn't directly absorbed in the body since it has to be bound to another substance in order for it to be absorbed. Thus, when looking for magnesium supplements, look for that form that is easily assimilated into the digestive system. The following are common forms of magnesium:

1. Magnesium Orotate

This is one of the most efficient types of magnesium and is made through the reaction of magnesium and mineral salts of Orotic acid. Both animal and plants use the Orotate in the synthesis of RNA and DNA, as they can penetrate most cell membranes. An Orotate is easily absorbed into the deepest layers of the nucleus and mitochondria cells. This form has many properties that can support health while still offering the cells the most absorbable magnesium variety.

2. Magnesium Citrate

This variety comes from magnesium salt reacting with citric acid and has a slightly lower concentration of magnesium. However, magnesium citrate has a very high bioavailability of over 90 percent hence is used for preventing kidney stones and to induce bowel movement.

3. Magnesium Amino Acid Chelate

This type of magnesium contains an ion of magnesium that is connected to a combination of magnesium and amino acids. The amino acids could be that of arginate, aspartate, glycine, or lactate. The most recommended form of chelated magnesium should be that of arginate or aspartate amino acid.

4. Magnesium Lactate

This lactate form of magnesium has moderate concentration, though has a higher assimilation level. This variety is used to address digestive problems, but should be avoided if suffering from kidney diseases.

5. Magnesium Sulfate

This inorganic magnesium has around 10 percent of magnesium and low level of assimilation or bioavailability. It contains magnesium element, oxygen, and sulfur and is also known as Epsom Salt.

6. Magnesium Carbonate

The carbonate form of magnesium has moderate amounts of magnesium element and has an assimilation rate of around 30 percent. The carbonate has higher levels of laxative, especially when consumed in high amounts. This form is also referred to as chalk and is mostly used as a drying agent by weight lifters, rock climbers, gymnasts, and pitchers.

7. Magnesium Taurates, Glycinate, & Malate

These three forms of magnesium have moderate to low concentrations of elemental composition but with high bioavailability levels. The varieties have multiple uses though they are not as essential as other forms of magnesium.

8. Magnesium Oxide

This form is also termed as "Magnesia", and is applied in therapeutic uses as a relief for acid reflux and as a laxative. Magnesium oxide is a highly concentrated form of magnesium but has lower levels of bioavailability of about 4 percent. The term bioavailability is used to describe the assimilation level of a mineral into the blood, bones, or other body tissues.

The key point about intake of magnesium is taking it in combination with calcium, thus look for supplements with sufficient levels of calcium and magnesium Orotate.

Now that you understand the different forms of magnesium that you can take in case of need for supplementation, let us look at importance of magnesium in our bodies with great emphasis on importance of magnesium in women's health.

IMPORTANCE OF MAGNESIUM TO WOMEN'S HEALTH

Everyone needs magnesium for various body functions such as for building stronger bones, boosting your mood, dealing with depression, treating respiratory disorders and gastrointestinal issues. However, of the two genders, women need magnesium in a higher supply compared to men especially in supporting pregnancy, dealing with headaches, anxiety, PMS and other related problems that affect the majority of women. Let's see how magnesium is important for women:

Magnesium for Pregnancy
When pregnant, you require sufficient amounts of magnesium to help protect against various problems such a preterm delivery and preeclampsia. Preeclampsia is a pregnancy complication that affects around 5 percent of women and is characterized by hypertension. The other feature of the condition is damage of the blood vessels of the kidneys, lungs, liver, or brain and can result to multiple organ failure followed by convulsions then coma and death. This condition is only cured through the delivery of the child.

Other problems related to pregnancy that magnesium can help prevent is poor fetal growth and infant mortality. It is advisable for a pregnant woman aged 19-30 years to consume around 350 grams of magnesium per day.

Magnesium for PMS

Magnesium is used in multiple enzymatic reactions that regulate the functioning of the brain and help relief disorders such as bipolar and PMS. Magnesium is also useful in relieving muscle cramps or the spasms, in the production of energy and in boosting proper functioning of the heart. It is advisable to increase magnesium intake at the onset of your menstrual flow in order to control severe mood changes.

Lowers Risk of Diabetes

Scientific research has established that overweight women who were taking a little amount of magnesium are more exposed to type II diabetes. The study involving around 40000 women recommended that women should take higher levels of magnesium by consuming foods like almonds and fresh veggies as well as supplementation.

Lowers Blood Pressure

Medical experts recommend a sufficient intake of magnesium to lower blood pressure. Based on a number of research studies, women are advised to consume a high dietary amount of magnesium in order to lower the risk of hypertension, especially during pregnancy. Why is this so, you may ask? Magnesium plays an important role in expanding the blood vessels and thus reduces the pressure of blood, to ease problems such as eclampsia and preeclampsia. Both of these conditions result in a sharp rise in blood pressure during the third trimester.

Magnesium has also been proven to work effectively and prevent other problems such as seizures. If you are a woman aged around 31 years and above, you should aim to consume about 320mg of magnesium.

Relieves Leg Cramps

Many pregnant women experience painful leg cramps. The condition can effectively be prevented through a 3-week intake of magnesium supplements.

Prevents Osteoporosis

Bone health is basically enhanced through the intake of calcium, vitamin D, and magnesium. Women achieve their peak bone mass when between 18-30 years, after which there's a gradual loss of bone density. During menopause, there is even accelerated the rate of bone loss. Lack of sufficient magnesium has shown to cause postmenopausal osteoporosis. This condition normally occurs in pregnant women during menopausal years and is characterized by extremely porous bones that can easily fracture. This condition is brought about by the fact that deficiency of magnesium can alter the metabolism of calcium and the hormones that monitor calcium.

Prevents Stress Attack

Are you aware that sufficient magnesium can help you overcome stress attacks and heal your nervous system? In addition to treating insomnia and depression, magnesium can help relieve other severe forms of psychiatric dysfunctions among them undue agitations and panic attacks.

Prevents Cardiovascular Diseases and Diabetes

It is advisable for women to consume magnesium rich foods and supplements in order to lower the risk of coronary heart diseases. A number of dietary surveys have concluded that taking sufficient amounts of magnesium can lower chances of getting a stroke. On the other hand, low magnesium level increases risks of getting a heart attack. Therefore, try getting enough of magnesium to improve your cardiovascular health.

In addition to the deficiency of magnesium causing cardiovascular disease, lack of magnesium can cause type II diabetes along with severe diabetic retinopathy. This is because magnesium is involved in the metabolism of carbohydrates and influences the production and functioning of insulin. Intake of around 100mg of magnesium can lower the risk of diabetes by 15 percent.

I am sure you know now how important it is especially for women to take magnesium. So, what would happen if you don't take adequate amounts of magnesium and thus suffer from magnesium deficiency?

CONDITIONS RELATED TO MAGNESIUM DEFICIENCY

Basically, there's no laboratory testing that can establish the correct amount of magnesium in your body tissues. This is because only 1% of the mineral is distributed into your blood serum, thus complicating the testing process. Doctors often try the urine tests to evaluate magnesium levels, but such tests only show estimated results.

Usually, the amount of magnesium in your body is mostly evaluated alongside the symptoms that you exhibit. Insufficient of magnesium may not necessarily cause you to experience any particular symptoms, but a full-blown deficiency of magnesium can make you feel weak, fatigued, and nauseated. Severe deficiency can cause serious problems such as abnormal heart rhythm, seizures, muscle contractions, tingling, and numbness, as well as involuntary eye movements.

You may also experience chronic symptoms such as coronary spasm, an effect that is characterized by blockage of blood flow of the arteries through which blood is supplied to the heart. Greater deficiency of magnesium can cause hypocalcemia or low calcium and low potassium or hypokalemia, fatal conditions. Severely low amounts of magnesium in the body can lead to respiratory arrest, heart attack, and death.

The following are conditions associated with deficiency in magnesium.

Atherosclerosis

This cardiovascular infection is characterized by clogging and hardening of the arteries or other blood vessels. The condition is basically caused by the accumulation of fatty acids deposits or cholesterol. Insufficient amounts of magnesium can worsen the condition as it interferes with metabolism, blood pressure, and platelet aggregation. Normally, deficiency in magnesium results to increased levels of bad cholesterol, reduced levels of HDL or good cholesterol, and more triglycerides. Consumption of magnesium can help reduce the bad LDL cholesterol while increase the levels of good HDL fatty acids.

Osteoporosis

Scientific studies show that the increase in levels of magnesium intake can boost the density of your bones by 80 percent. If you are a woman experiencing post menopause, you need to consume at least 1000mg of calcium daily in order to increase the dietary magnesium to calcium ratio. The recommended ratio of the two minerals is 1:2, but women should consume more calcium to make the ratio 1:4.

Asthma

A number of studies have found that in case you suffer from asthma, your magnesium content is usually low, and that boosting of magnesium can relief asthma symptoms. Supplementation with magnesium has shown improved activity of the lung and the ability to circulate air in and out of the lungs. On the other hand, insufficient levels of magnesium result into aggravated asthmatic conditions and reported wheezing.

Most multivitamins do not contain magnesium, as the mineral is quite bulky and can make the tablet quite large. Others contain magnesium antagonists that work to reduce the amount of magnesium level in the body. That is why continued usage of multivitamins is associated with the development of asthma and allergies.

Calcification

This condition can be described as a change into stony or calcareous substance through the deposit of lime or calcium salt. The condition may occur in the kidney as well as in heart valves. Renal calculi are characterized by the deposit of calcium phosphate salts into the kidney, an organ that filters the blood and produces urine. Oral intake of magnesium has shown to reduce the formation of stones or urine saturation index. On the other hand, magnesium deficiency can cause calcification of human heart valves. Intake of magnesium as an oral therapy has also proved to reduce the condition.

Attention Deficit Disorder

Are you aware that the main causes of Attention Deficit Hyperactivity Disorder (ADHD) and Attention Deficit Disorder (ADD) is magnesium deficiency? Research has shown that lack of sufficient magnesium is one of the main causes of the conditions. About 95 percent of children who suffer from the two attention deficit disorders are magnesium deficient.

Diabetes

Magnesium deficiency is attributed to worsening the cases of diabetes, which is the 7th leading cause of death among Americans. Most people do not consume the required amounts of magnesium and thus are at risk of getting type II diabetes. The best sources of magnesium are magnesium rich food as supplements and multivitamins are not as effective on diabetes.

Anxiety and Psychiatric Disorders

There is a direct link between magnesium consumption and anxiety and depression disorders. Deficiency of this vital mineral often leads to an increase in depression and anxiety in a majority of people. Lack of magnesium in the blood serum can also lead to a state of enhanced anxiety and hyperactivity. It is important to note that your body requires magnesium in order to transport adrenaline in the body, to control hypertension and to relax the contracted muscles. A deficiency in magnesium, therefore, results to tense muscles, high blood pressure, and excess amounts of adrenaline that contributes to hyperactivity.

Allergies

Deficiency of magnesium has shown adverse allergic reactions and chemical sensitivities, a condition that is characterized by increased scratching, and skin redness. With allergic reactions, the levels of histamine and white blood cells also increase. When suffering from chronic disorders, you tend to have skin allergies, raised white blood cells level, and other varied types of allergies.

With the information obtained about conditions that you can suffer due to magnesium deficiency, then it is critical to fighting magnesium deficiency. Let us see how we can use diet to achieve that.

USING DIET TO FIGHT MAGNESIUM DEFICIENCY

Once you realize that you suffer from magnesium deficiency, you need to consume the mineral from the whole foods that contain it in organic form. Plants contain the green coloring mater known as chlorophyll, which is useful in converting energy from the sun into metabolic energy. The chlorophyll is composed of magnesium and it's the mineral that allows the plant to absorb solar energy. Green veggies among them Swiss chard and spinach are rich sources of magnesium, as well as beans and avocados. Other sources are nuts and seeds such as sesame seeds, sunflower seeds, pumpkin seeds, and almonds.

In as much as you need to take foods rich in magnesium, you may also want to note that some conditions or factors can affect the absorption of magnesium and thus may render you deficient even after consumption. Thus in order to be sure you are taking sufficient levels, you need to confirm the following problems don't interfere with magnesium uptake and utilization. They include:

1. Unhealthy digestive system, which can inhibit your body's ability to absorb magnesium, due to problems among them leaky gut or Crohn's disease

2. Infected kidneys which cause excess loss of magnesium through urination

3. Diabetes disease, particularly when not controlled, which

leads to increase in loss of magnesium through urination

4. Various medications, among them antibiotics, diuretics and other medications used in treating cancer. These conditions can result into a deficiency of magnesium.

5. Alcoholism, in which more than 60 percent of alcoholics have very low levels of magnesium

6. Age, as older people have a higher chance of being magnesium deficient as the rate of absorption reduces with age. The elderly women are also likely to take more medications, which then interfere with the absorption of magnesium.

7. Candida, which can prevent your body from absorption of magnesium since high levels of Candida in the body utilize magnesium to break down the Candida metabolites, resulting into a deficiency

8. A daily drinker of caffeinated drinks among them soda, tea, and coffee, since kidneys monitor magnesium levels and caffeine makes the kidneys release magnesium regardless of your body condition

FOODS WITH HIGH MAGNESIUM LEVEL

It is more advisable to control magnesium levels through nutrition instead of using supplements. One of the easiest ways is to eat a varied diet that incorporates many dark-green leafy veggies that are grown organically. Plants grew using fertilizers often have high amounts of potassium, phosphorus and nitrogen as opposed to magnesium. This list shows some of the 8 most magnesium-rich foods based on the magnesium content in every 100 grams:

Dried seaweed that contains 770 mg magnesium
Dried coriander leaf, 694 mg
Dried pumpkin seeds, containing 535 mg
Dry powdered and unsweetened Cocoa with 499 mg
Dried Basil, with 422 mg
Ground Flaxseed, 392 mg
Almond butter, about 303 mg
Sweet and dried whey with 176 mg

The following are varieties of food choices that you should choose to obtain your much-needed magnesium content.

Dark Leafy Greens
These are very vital super foods, which offer a number of essential vitamins and minerals along with other health benefits. Dark leafy greens serve as better choices for magnesium source as they are also not high in calories. The best greens to go for include

Swiss chard, kale, collard greens, raw or baby spinach.

Nuts and Seeds
Do you know just half a cup of pumpkin seeds almost offers your entire daily magnesium nutritional requirement? Other nuts that are rich in magnesium include pecans, flaxseeds, pine nuts, cashews, Brazil nuts, sunflower seeds, and almonds.

Fish
In addition to the high amounts of vitamin D and omega 3 fatty acids, you should add more fish into your diet to obtain magnesium. Fish such as tuna, halibut, wild salmon, and mackerel have high levels of the mineral. Ensure that you consume fish for lunch or dinner once per week, or a try making a salmon salad.

Soybeans
This legume is rich in nutrients such as amino acids, vitamins, and minerals and has high amounts of fiber. Soybeans nearly offer half of your daily magnesium requirement. Aim for ½ cup serving of dry and roasted soybeans as your snack, to benefit from these nutrients. Other legumes also have high amounts of magnesium. They include lentils, black-eyed peas, chickpeas, white beans, kidney beans, and black beans.

Avocado
This fruit is high in heart healthy nutrients as well as various multivitamins and is actually one of the most nutritious and versatile foods you can eat. Incorporate a sliced avocado into your sandwich for lunch, or make into a salad to obtain 15 percent of the daily-required content of magnesium.

Bananas
Bananas are famous for their ample amounts of potassium that work to strengthen your bones and promote heart health. Additionally, a medium sized banana can offer you around 32 milligrams of magnesium along with vitamin C and fiber. Therefore, a banana is a good choice for dieters as it only contains 100 calories, and thus should be a part of your breakfast or snack.

Other fruits that equally have high amounts of magnesium include figs, grape fruit, blackberries, and strawberries.

Dark Chocolate

In addition to its sweet taste, dark chocolate is a good choice for a daily snack or dessert as it contains high amounts of magnesium. A square of dark chocolate offers around 24 percent of the daily recommended magnesium and is not high in calorie as it only contains 145 calories. Dark chocolate is also rich in antioxidants that can relief hypertension, boost heart health, and improve blood circulation. Try pairing dark chocolate with a fresh fruit to constitute sweet and delicious after-dinner desert.

Low-Fat Yogurt

For your body to absorb magnesium, you also need to factor in calcium as part of the nutritional content. Dairy products among them yogurt are a great source of magnesium too. A container of low or no-fat yogurt contains around 19 milligrams of magnesium. Try incorporating a fiber-rich fruit with low-fat yogurt for your breakfast.

DIETARY TIPS TO INCREASE MAGNESIUM INTAKE

1. Aim for more magnesium-rich meals among them veggies, nuts, and beans. Veggies are very suitable for dieters aiming to burn fat or lose weight as they contain fewer calories. Try making a soup from veggies, meat, and beans, simmer it overnight in your Crockpot and consume the following morning for breakfast.

2. Try eating healthy fats along with your diet in order to boost the absorption of nutrients. Scientific research has proven that magnesium is easily absorbed with consumption of salad containing fat.

3. While you need to take in adequate amounts of calcium to ensure adequate absorption of magnesium, too much calcium is not good. Therefore, avoid eating too much calcium rich foods or drinking excess milk as this might lower magnesium level in the body. In addition, taking calcium in large amounts interferes with proper functioning of your heart which magnesium tries to enhance.

4. Try obtaining magnesium from dietary sources as opposed to supplements, as magnesium is an alkaline mineral. Supplementing with magnesium lowers your stomach's acidity and thus hinders nutrient absorption. You also need other minerals for proper assimilation as opposed to supplements that offer only magnesium.

5. Do not consume soy products in excess as they raise estrogen levels and thus hinder absorption and utilization of magnesium in your body. Soy foods can also result to thyroid problems and thus should be consumed in moderation.

.

.

USING SUPPLEMENTS TO FIGHT DEFICIENCY

Magnesium deficiency problems that supplements are designed to address include migraine headaches, kidney stones and hearing loss. Magnesium supplements are also believed to cure insomnia, restless leg syndrome and enhance athletic performance.

Medical experts in most circumstances may recommend you to use supplements to treat problems such as premenstrual syndrome (PMS), eclampsia, preeclampsia, hypertension or a very high level of high-density lipoprotein or bad cholesterol. You can also be required to buy magnesium supplements to address chronic conditions such as chronic fatigue syndrome, fibromyalgia, multiple sclerosis, and diabetes. In rare cases, magnesium supplements can be used for asthma, altitude sickness, chronic obstructive pulmonary disease (COPD) and Lyme disease.

Across the two genders, the older adults seem to have a lower level of magnesium compared to younger adults. This is caused by the inability of the gut to absorb magnesium as well as the kidney being unable to retain magnesium as you age. In case you suffer from type II diabetes, your kidney may excrete a lot of magnesium causing its deficit.

Do magnesium supplements work?
It's believed that supplementing with magnesium tablets can

raise the level of magnesium in the blood serum and bones. The most effective form of magnesium supplements is those in the form of chloride, lactate, citrate, and aspartate. According to a number of research studies, people taking the supplements end up having more than the recommended daily allowance. The recommended amount of magnesium should be within 320-420 milligrams daily, which depends on the age or the activity.

Long-term studies have shown a connection between the high level of magnesium and a reduced risk of developing a heart disease, ischemic heart disease, stroke, and sudden cardiac death.

In about 7 studies that were done to more than 200, 000 participants, it was found that about 100 milligrams in excess magnesium daily can reduce your risk of stroke by around 8 percent. Though magnesium supplements are believed to lower hypertension, the effectiveness is not as it seems to be. Around 22 studies conducted on magnesium and hypertension found out that magnesium only managed to lower the pressure by 2-4 mmHg. Actually, hypertension can be as high with 20 mmHg, increasing from 140/90mmHg to 160/100 mmHg. The analysis to these studies indicated that hypertension was effectively addressed through an increase in magnesium content from fruits and veggies.

Supplements should offer at least 370 mg of magnesium daily to be effective, against the recommended 320 mg daily. Using of fruits and veggies also boosts the levels of other nutrients such as calcium or potassium. Thus, it is hard to determine independently how magnesium affects high blood pressure when the diet is used in place of supplements.

Type II diabetes is linked to low magnesium levels as deficiency of the mineral worsens insulin resistance, which results to unmonitored levels of blood sugar. However, insulin resistance can also cause a deficiency of magnesium, thus it's difficult to establish how the two affect each other. Diabetes may cause low levels of magnesium, which will cause the worsening of diabetes. On the other hand, magnesium supplements have shown potential in preventing migraine. However, a nutritional supplement butterbur is more advised for migraine prevention as compared to the use of magnesium.

More studies with the National Library of Medicine have found that magnesium supplements can help address pain from fibromyalgia and chronic fatigue syndrome. There's also evidence that they can assist in treating PMS, asthma attacks, hearing loss, kidney stones, high cholesterol and Chronic Obstructive Pulmonary Disease. However, there isn't enough studies to establish whether supplements may help address problems such as multiple sclerosis or Lyme disease, hay fever, ADHD, and anxiety.

Are the supplements safe?
Magnesium remains one of the 7 major elements required in the body, and its deficiency can pose serious problems among them death. On the other hand, taking in excess of one mineral can lead to a deficiency of another, where excessive magnesium generally causes a deficiency in calcium. It is quite hard to overdose magnesium from an ordinary diet, and overdose generally happens from laxatives or supplements.

If you suffer from kidney problems, you're more likely to face an overdose of magnesium. Consumption of magnesium to toxic levels can lead to symptoms such as diarrhea and stomach upsets, to other serious conditions like low blood pressure, slowed heart rate, confusion, and vomiting. A more severe overdose of magnesium can cause irregular heartbeat, coma, and problems in breathing or even death.

Additionally, magnesium supplements may interfere with other drugs among them antibiotics meant to address bacterial infections. The supplements can cause low absorption of antibiotics such as moxifloxacin and ciprofloxacin. The supplements are also counteractive on with osteoporosis drugs if taken too close, and can interfere with medications meant to address thyroid problems.

Magnesium may also worsen the side effects of hypertension medications and raise the potency of diabetes medicines.

With all the information on magnesium, its deficiency and using diet and supplements to deal with deficiency, it is important to look at ways of addressing magnesium deficiency for long term health.

ELIMINATING MAGNESIUM DEFICIENCY FOR LONG-TERM

Insufficient magnesium can lead to many health problems among them immune system depression, disrupted recovery and sleep, lack of energy, excess soreness, and muscle cramping. During intense activity, the deficiency can lead to fatal heart arrhythmias or irregular heartbeat. Magnesium is usually important in buffering the lactic acid and enhances uptake of oxygen and total work output. This reduces the heart rate and generation of carbon dioxide when doing tough exercises, and improves efficiency in cardiovascular activity.

Veggies, grains, nuts, and seeds can offer high amounts of magnesium, especially for active women. However, you can still be magnesium deficient even if you include these foods into the diets due to the combination of mineral loss through perspiration. Additionally, if you have an active lifestyle, you also face an accelerated mineral turn over that may cause depletion. In such cases, use of oral magnesium supplements may not completely deal with deficiency, as the amount of magnesium taken orally is not easily absorbed. Trying to take higher dosages of magnesium will definitely make the condition worse.

A better way of addressing deficiency of magnesium is through a technique referred as the transdermal application. Deficiency of magnesium can be addressed through the skin, a practice that is done in place of intravenous therapies. Applying magnesium through the skin can be effective in improving the absorption as the supplement travels through the gastrointestinal tract. The method also helps lower the metabolism of the drug by the liver and provides a more targeted application.

This method of application can also be used to deliver high dosages of precisely targeted magnesium supplement through the muscles before or after a workout. This treatment is aimed at boosting the performance and the recovery. As this transdermal magnesium bypasses the process of digestion, it's easier to achieve higher doses of the mineral as targeted. However, you need to monitor the amount of magnesium taken through transdermal delivery, as more than 500-1000 mg of magnesium can lead to health problems.

A way of using transdermal magnesium application is for instance trying an Epsom salt bath to deal with muscle soreness. Epsom salts deliver magnesium sulfate, to help address post workout recovery though more benefits can come from magnesium chloride crystals or flakes in the bath. Doing a magnesium chloride flake bath should deliver around 500mg of magnesium. In case you don't wish to hop into a full bath, you can as well soak your feet in magnesium chloride footbath especially after a long run or ride.

You can also enjoy benefits of topical magnesium that is also available as a form of spray, which you can use a number of sprays before workout. For instance, you can spray about 8-10 times on each arm, leg, or shoulders before a race or hard activity for longevity and optimal performance.

Therefore, your goal is to ensure that you take foods rich in magnesium, embrace supplementation, and topical use of magnesium for long term health and longevity.

CONCLUSION

Magnesium is very important for the proper functioning of your body especially for pregnant women. In order to increase your magnesium levels, it is important to eat foods that are high in magnesium as opposed to supplementation. However, if you still suffer from magnesium deficiency even after taking adequate amounts of magnesium, you could be having an absorption problem and you should look at the problems I highlighted in an earlier chapter that can cause magnesium deficiency despite taking the require amounts of magnesium. Correct the problem and increase magnesium levels in your body.

Thank you and good luck!

Kara Aimer

ADDITIONAL RESOURCES

Please point your web browser to **www.plaid-enterprises.com** for more related resources, my full bibliography and to grab your FREE book!

www.ingramcontent.com/pod-product-compliance
Lightning Source LLC
Chambersburg PA
CBHW070938290526
45795CB00003B/1070